My Vibrant Keto Chaffle Cookbook

50 Creative Keto Chaffle Ideas for your Lifestyle

Imogene Cook

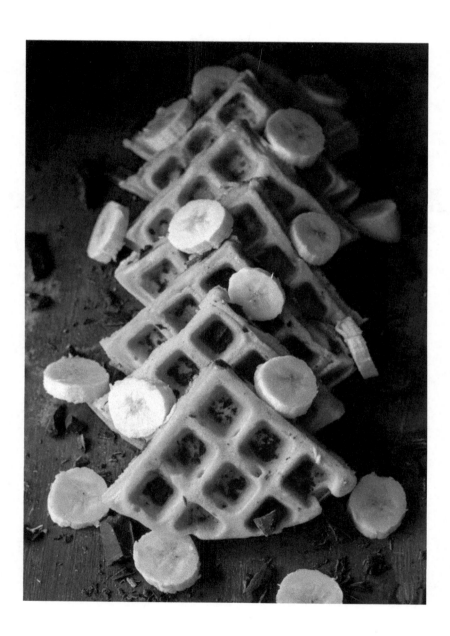

How to Make Chaffles?

Equipment and Ingredients Discussed

Making chaffles requires five simple steps and nothing more than a waffle maker for flat chaffles and a waffle bowl maker for chaffle bowls.

To make chaffles, you will need two necessary ingredients –eggs and cheese. My preferred cheeses are cheddar cheese or mozzarella cheese. These melt quickly, making them the go-to for most recipes. Meanwhile, always ensure that your cheeses are finely grated or thinly sliced for use.

Now, to make a standard chaffle:

First, preheat your waffle maker until adequately hot.

Meanwhile, in a bowl, mix the egg with cheese on hand until well combined.

Open the iron, pour in a quarter or half of the mixture, and close.

Cook the chaffle for 5 to 7 minutes or until it is crispy.

Transfer the chaffle to a plate and allow cooling before serving.

11 Tips to Make Chaffles

My surefire ways to turn out the crispiest of chaffles:

Preheat Well: Yes! It sounds obvious to preheat the waffle iron before usage. However, preheating the iron moderately

 will not get your chaffles as crispy as you will like. The best way to preheat before cooking is to ensure that the iron is very hot.

Not-So-Cheesy: Will you prefer to have your chaffles less cheesy? Then use mozzarella cheese.

Not-So Eggy: If you aren't comfortable with the smell of eggs in your chaffles, try using egg whites instead of egg yolks or whole eggs.

 To Shred or to Slice: Many recipes call for shredded cheese when making chaffles, but I find sliced cheeses to offer crispier pieces. While I stick with mostly shredded cheese for convenience's sake, be at ease to use sliced cheese in the same quantity. When using sliced cheeses, arrange two to four pieces in the waffle iron, top with the beaten eggs, and some slices of the cheese. Cover and cook until crispy.

Shallower Irons: For better crisps on your chaffles, use shallower waffle irons as they cook easier and faster.

Layering: Don't fill up the waffle iron with too much batter. Work between a quarter and a half cup of total ingredients per batch for correctly done chaffles.

Patience: It is a virtue even when making chaffles. For the best results, allow the chaffles to sit in the iron for 5 to 7 minutes before serving.

No Peeking: 7 minutes isn't too much of a time to wait for the outcome of your chaffles, in my opinion.

Opening the iron and checking on the chaffle before

it is done stands you a worse chance of ruining it.

Crispy Cooling: For better crisp, I find that allowing the chaffles to cool further after they are transferred to a plate aids a lot.

Easy Cleaning: For the best cleanup, wet a paper towel and wipe the inner parts of the iron clean while still warm. Kindly note that the iron should be warm but not hot!

Brush It: Also, use a clean toothbrush to clean between the iron's teeth for a thorough cleanup. You may also use a dry, rough sponge to clean the iron while it is still warm.

Choco And Strawberries Chaffles

Preparation time: 10 minutes

Cooking Time: 5 minutes

Servings: 2

Ingredients:

- 1 tbsp. almond flour
- 1/2 cup strawberry puree
- 1/2 cup cheddar cheese
- 1 tbsp. cocoa powder
- ½ tsp baking powder
- 1 large egg
- 2 tbsps. coconut oil. melted
- 1/2 tsp vanilla extract optional

Directions:

1. Preheat waffle iron while you are mixing the ingredients.
2. Melt oil in a microwave.
3. In a small mixing bowl, mix together flour, baking powder, flour, and vanilla until well combined.

4. Add egg, melted oil, ½ cup cheese and strawberry puree to the flour mixture.

5. Pour 1/8 cup cheese in a waffle maker and then pour the mixture in the center of greased waffle.

6. Again, sprinkle cheese on the batter.

7. Close the waffle maker.

8. Cook chaffles for about 4-5 minutes Utes until cooked and crispy.

9. Once chaffles are cooked, remove and enjoy!

Nutrition:

Protein: 15% 48 kcal Fat: 79% 246 kcal Carbohydrates: 5% 17 kcal

Lemon and Paprika Chaffles

Preparation time: 8 minutes

Cooking Time: 28 Minutes

Servings: 2

Ingredients:

- 1 egg, beaten
- 1 oz cream cheese, softened
- 1/3 cup finely grated mozzarella cheese
- 1 tbsp almond flour
- 1 tsp butter, melted
- 1 tsp maple (sugar-free) syrup
- ½ tsp sweet paprika
- ½ tsp lemon extract

Directions:

1. Preheat the waffle iron.
2. Mix all the ingredients in a medium bowl
3. Open the iron and pour in a quarter of the mixture. Close and cook until crispy, 7 minutes.

4. Remove the chaffle onto a plate and make 3 more with the remaining mixture.

5. Cut each chaffle into wedges, plate, allow cooling and serve.

Nutrition:

Calories 48 Fats 4.22g Carbs 0.Net Carbs 0.5g Protein 2g

Triple Chocolate Chaffle

Preparation time: 5 minutes

Cooking Time:7–9 Minutes

Servings: 2

Ingredients:

Batter

- 4 eggs
- 4 ounces cream cheese, softened
- 1 ounce dark unsweetened chocolate, melted
- 1 teaspoon vanilla extract
- 5 tablespoons almond flour
- 3 tablespoons cocoa powder
- 1½ teaspoons baking powder
- ¼ cup dark unsweetened chocolate chips Other
- 2 tablespoons butter to brush the waffle maker

Directions:

1. Preheat the waffle maker.

2. Add the eggs and cream cheese to a bowl and stir with a wire whisk until just combined.
3. Add the vanilla extract and mix until combined.
4. Stir in the almond flour, cocoa powder, and baking powder and mix until combined.
5. Add the chocolate chips and stir.
6. Brush the heated waffle maker with butter and add a few tablespoons of the batter.
7. Close the lid and cook for about 8 minutes depending on your waffle maker.
8. Serve and enjoy.

Nutrition:

Calories 385, fat 33 g, carbs 10.6 g, sugar 0.7 g, Protein 12.g, sodium 199 mg

Basic Chaffle

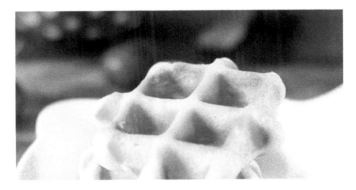

Preparation time: 10 minutes

Cooking Time: 8 Minutes

Servings: 2

Ingredients:

- Cooking spray
- 1 egg
- ½ cup cheddar cheese, shredded

Directions:

1. Turn your waffle maker on.
2. Grease both sides with cooking spray.
3. Beat the egg in a bowl.
4. Stir in the cheddar cheese.

---

5. Pour half of the batter into the waffle maker.

6. Seal and cook for 4 minutes.

7. Remove the chaffle slowly from the waffle maker.

8. Let sit for 3 minutes.

9. Pour the remaining batter into the waffle maker and repeat the steps.

Nutrition:

Calories 191 Total Fat 23 g Saturated Fat 14 g Cholesterol 223 mg Sodium 413 mg Potassium 116 mg Total Carbohydrate 1 g Dietary Fiber 1 g Protein 20 g Total Sugars 1 g

Nut Butter Chaffle

Preparation time: 10 minutes

Cooking Time: 8 Minutes

Servings: 2

Ingredients:

- 1 egg
- ½ cup mozzarella cheese, shredded
- 2 tablespoons almond flour
- ½ teaspoon baking powder
- 1 tablespoon sweetener
- 1 teaspoon vanilla
- 2 tablespoons nut butter

Directions:

1. Turn on the waffle maker.
2. Beat the egg in a bowl and combine with the cheese.
3. In another bowl, mix the almond flour, baking powder and sweetener.
4. In the third bowl, blend the vanilla extract and nut butter.

5. Gradually add the almond flour mixture into the egg mixture.
6. Then, stir in the vanilla extract.
7. Pour the batter into the waffle maker.
8. Cook for 4 minutes.
9. Transfer to a plate and let cool for 2 minutes.
10. Repeat the steps with the remaining batter.

Nutrition:

Calories 168 Total Fat 15.5g Saturated Fat 3.9g Cholesterol 34mg Sodium 31mg Potassium 64mg Total Carbohydrate 1.6gDietary Fiber 1.4g Protein 5.4g Total Sugars 0.6g

Keto Coffee Chaffles

Preparation time: 10 minutes

Cooking Time: 5 minutes

Servings: 2

Ingredients:

- 1 tbsp. almond flour
- 1 tbsp. instant coffee
- 1/2 cup cheddar cheese
- ½ tsp baking powder
- 1 large egg

Directions:

1. Preheat waffle iron and grease with cooking spray
2. Meanwhile, in a small mixing bowl, mix together all ingredients and ½ cup cheese.
3. Pour 1/8 cup cheese in a waffle maker and then pour the mixture in the center of greased waffle.
4. Again, sprinkle cheese on the batter.
5. Close the waffle maker.

6. Cook chaffles for about 4-5 minutes Utes until cooked and crispy.
7. Once chaffles are cooked, remove and enjoy!

Nutrition:

Protein: 26% 47 kcal Fat: 69% 125 kcal Carbohydrates: 5% 9 kcal

Chaffle Ice Cream Bowl

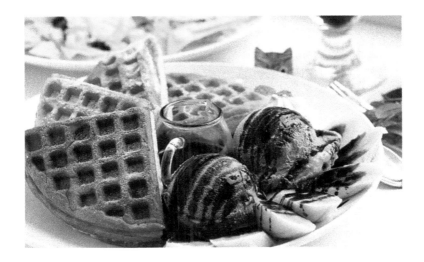

Preparation time: 10 minutes

Cooking Time: 0 Minutes

Servings: 2

Ingredients:

- 4 basic chaffles
- 2 scoops keto ice cream
- 2 teaspoons sugar-free chocolate syrup

Directions:

1. Arrange 2 basic chaffles in a bowl, following the contoured design of the bowl.
2. Top with the ice cream.
3. Drizzle with the syrup on top.
4. Serve.

Nutrition: Calories 181 Total Fat 17.2g Saturated Fat4.2g Cholesterol26mg Sodium 38mg Total Carbohydrate 7g Dietary Fiber 1g Total Sugars 4.1g Protein 0.4g Potassium 0mg

Peanut Butter Sandwich Chaffle

Preparation time: 10 minutes

Cooking Time: 15 Minutes

Servings: 2

Ingredients:

For chaffle:

- 1 egg, lightly beaten
- 1/2 cup mozzarella cheese, shredded
- 1/4 tsp espresso powder
- 1 tbsp unsweetened chocolate chips
- 1 tbsp Swerve
- 2 tbsp unsweetened cocoa powder

For filling:

- 1 tbsp butter, softened
- 2 tbsp Swerve
- 3 tbsp creamy peanut butter

Directions:

1. Preheat your waffle maker.
2. In a bowl, whisk together egg, espresso powder, chocolate chips, Swerve, and cocoa powder.
3. Add mozzarella cheese and stir well.
4. Spray waffle maker with cooking spray.
5. Pour 1/2 of the batter in the hot waffle maker and cook for 3-4 minutes or until golden brown. Repeat with the remaining batter.
6. For filling: In a small bowl, stir together butter, Swerve, and peanut butter until smooth.
7. Once chaffles is cool, then spread filling mixture between two chaffle and place in the fridge for 10 minutes.
8. Cut chaffle sandwich in half and serve.

Nutrition:

Calories 1 Fat 16.1 carbohydrates 9.6 sugar 1.1 protein 8.2

cholesterol 101 mg

Chocolate Chaffle Rolls

Preparation time: 7 minutes

Cooking Time: 10 Minutes

Servings: 2

Ingredients:

- 1/2 cup mozzarella cheese
- 1 tbsp. almond flour
- 1 egg
- 1 tsp cinnamon
- 1 tsp stevia

FILLING

- 1 tbsp. coconut cream
- 1 tbsp. coconut flour
- 1/4 cup keto chocolate chips

Directions:

1. Switch on a round waffle maker and let it heat up.

2. In a small bowl, mix together cheese, egg, flour, cinnamon powder, and stevia in a bowl.
3. Spray the round waffle maker with nonstick spray.
4. Pour the batter in a waffle maker and close the lid.
5. Close the waffle maker and cook for about 3-4 minutes Utes.
6. Once chaffles are cooked remove from Maker
7. Meanwhile, mix together cream flour and chocolate chips in bowl and microwave for 30 sec.
8. Spread this filling over chaffle and roll it.
9. Serve and enjoy!

Nutrition:

Protein: 32% 50 kcal Fat: 61% 94 kcal Carbohydrates: 7% 11 kcal

Chaffles Ice-cream Topping

Preparation time: 7 minutes

Cooking Time: 5 Minutes

Servings: 2

Ingredients:

- 1/4 cup coconut cream, frozen
- 1 cup coconut flour
- ¼ cup strawberries chunks
- 1 tsp. vanilla extract
- 1 oz. chocolate flakes
- 4 keto chaffles

Directions:

1. Mix together all ingredients in a mixing bowl.
2. Spread mixture between chaffles and freeze in the freezer for 2 hours.
3. Serve chill and enjoy!

Nutrition: Protein: 26% 68 kcal Fat: 71% 187 kcal Carbohydrates: 3% 9 kcal

Easter Morning Simple Chaffles

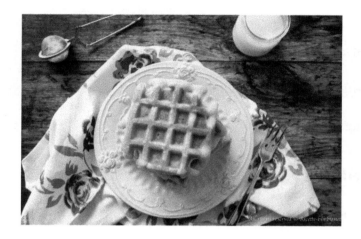

Preparation time: 7 minutes

Cooking Time: 5 minutes

Servings: 2

Ingredients:

- 1/2 cup egg whites
- 1 cup mozzarella cheese, melted

Directions:

1. Switch on your square waffle maker. Spray with non-stick spray.
2. Beat egg whites with beater, until fluffy and white.
3. Add cheese and mix well.
4. Pour batter in a waffle maker.
5. Close the maker and cook for about 3 minutes Utes.
6. Repeat with the remaining batter.
7. Remove chaffles from the maker.
8. Serve hot and enjoy!

Nutrition:

Protein: 36% 42 kcal Fat: 60% 71 kcal Carbohydrates: 4% 5 kcal

Pumpkin Cheesecake Chaffle

Preparation time: 10 minutes

Cooking Time: 15 Minutes

Servings: 2

Ingredients:

For chaffle:

- 1 egg
- 1/2 tsp vanilla
- 1/2 tsp baking powder, gluten-free
- 1/4 tsp pumpkin spice
- 1 tsp cream cheese, softened
- 2 tsp heavy cream
- 1 tbsp Swerve
- 1 tbsp almond flour
- 2 tsp pumpkin puree
- 1/2 cup mozzarella cheese, shredded

For filling:

- 1/4 tsp vanilla
- 1 tbsp Swerve

- 2 tbsp cream cheese

Directions:

1. Preheat your mini waffle maker.
2. In a small bowl, mix all chaffle ingredients.
3. Spray waffle maker with cooking spray.
4. Pour half batter in the hot waffle maker and cook for 3-5 minutes. Repeat with the remaining batter.
5. In a small bowl, combine all filling ingredients.
6. Spread filling mixture between two chaffles and place in the fridge for 10 minutes.
7. Serve and enjoy.

Nutrition:

Calories 107Fat 7.2 carbohydrates 5 sugar 0.7 protein 6.7

cholesterol 93 mg

Cinnamon Chaffle Rolls

Preparation time: 7 minutes

Cooking Time:10 Minutes

Servings: 2

Ingredients:

- 1/2 cup mozzarella cheese
- 1 tbsp. almond flour
- 1 egg
- 1 tsp cinnamon
- 1 tsp stevia

CINNAMON ROLL GLAZE

- 1 tbsp. butter
- 1 tbsp. cream cheese
- 1 tsp. cinnamon
- 1/4 tsp vanilla extract
- 1 tbsp. coconut flour

Directions:

1. Switch on a round waffle maker and let it heat up.
2. In a small bowl mix together cheese, egg, flour, cinnamon powder, and stevia in a bowl.
3. Spray the round waffle maker with nonstick spray.
4. Pour the batter in a waffle maker and close the lid.
5. Close the waffle maker and cook for about 3-4 minutes Utes.
6. Once chaffles are cooked, remove from Maker
7. Mix together butter, cream cheese, cinnamon, vanilla and coconut flour in a bowl.
8. Spread this glaze over chaffle and roll up.
9. Serve and enjoy!

Nutrition:

Protein: 25% 52 kcal Fat: 69% 142 kcal Carbohydrates: 7% 14 kcal

Double Chocolate Chaffles

Preparation time: 10 minutes

Cooking Time:5 minutes

Servings: 2

Ingredients:

- 1/4 cup unsweetened chocolate chips
- 2 tbsps. cocoa powder
- 1 cup egg whites
- 1 tsp. coffee powder
- 2 tbsps. almond flour
- 1/2 cup mozzarella cheese
- 1 tbsp. coconut milk
- 1 tsp. baking powder
- 1 tsp. stevia

Directions:

1. Switch on your Belgian chaffle maker.
2. Spray the waffle maker with cooking spray.

3. Beat egg whites with an electric beater until fluffy and white.
4. Add the rest of the ingredients to the egg whites and mix them again.
5. Pour batter in a greased waffle maker and make two fluffy chaffles.
6. Once chaffles are cooked, remove from the maker.
7. Serve with coconut cream, and berries
8. Enjoy!

Nutrition:

Protein: 52% kcal Fat: 39% 73 kcal Carbohydrates: 9% 17 kcal

Breakfast Peanut Butter Chaffle

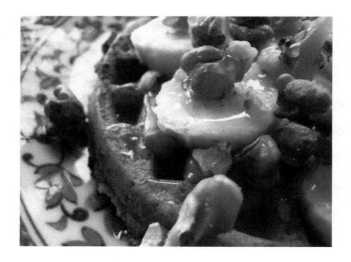

Preparation time: 10 minutes

Cooking Time: 15 Minutes

Servings: 2

Ingredients:

- 1 egg, lightly beaten
- ½ tsp vanilla
- 1 tbsp Swerve
- 2 tbsp powdered peanut butter
- ½ cup mozzarella cheese, shredded

Directions:

1. Preheat your waffle maker.
2. Add all ingredients into the bowl and mix until well combined.
3. Spray waffle maker with cooking spray.
4. Pour half batter in the hot waffle maker and cook for 5-7 minutes or until golden brown. Repeat with the remaining batter.
5. Serve and enjoy.

Nutrition:

Calories 80Fat 4.1 carbohydrates 2.9 sugar 0.g Protein 7.4 cholesterol 86 mg

Apple Cinnamon Chaffles

Preparation time: 6 minutes

Cooking Time: 20 Minutes

Servings: 2

Ingredients:

- 3 eggs, lightly beaten
- 1 cup mozzarella cheese, shredded
- ¼ cup apple, chopped
- ½ tsp monk fruit sweetener
- 1 ½ tsp cinnamon
- ¼ tsp baking powder, gluten-free
- 2 tbsp coconut flour

Directions:

1. Preheat your waffle maker.
2. Add remaining ingredients and stir until well combined.
3. Spray waffle maker with cooking spray.
4. Pour 1/3 of batter in the hot waffle maker and cook for minutes or until golden brown. Repeat with the

remaining batter.

5. Serve and enjoy.

Nutrition:

Calories 142Fat 7.4 carbohydrates 9.7 sugar 3 protein 9.g Cholesterol 169 mg

Churro Chaffle

Preparation time: 10 minutes

Cooking Time: 8 Minutes

Servings: 2

Ingredients:

- 1 egg
- ½ cup mozzarella cheese, shredded
- ½ teaspoon cinnamon
- 2 tablespoons sweetener

Directions:

1. Turn on your waffle iron.
2. Beat the egg in a bowl.
3. Stir in the cheese.
4. Pour half of the mixture into the waffle maker.
5. Cover the waffle iron.
6. Cook for 4 minutes.
7. While waiting, mix the cinnamon and sweetener in a bowl.

8. Open the device and soak the waffle in the cinnamon mixture.

9. Repeat the steps with the remaining batter.

Nutrition:

Calories Total Fat 6.9g Saturated Fat 2.9g Cholesterol 171mg Sodium 147mg Potassium 64mg Total Carbohydrate 5.8g Dietary Fiber 2.6g Protein 9.6g Total Sugars 0.4g

Blueberry Chaffles

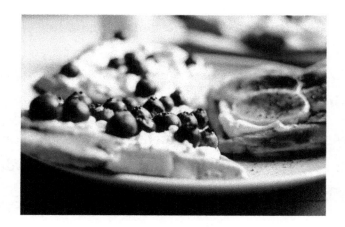

Preparation time: 8 minutes

Cooking Time: 15 Minutes

Servings: 2

Ingredients:

- 2 eggs
- 1/2 cup blueberries
- 1/2 tsp baking powder
- 1/2 tsp vanilla
- 2 tsp Swerve
- 3 tbsp almond flour
- 1 cup mozzarella cheese, shredded
-

Directions:

1. Preheat your waffle maker.
2. In a medium bowl, mix eggs, vanilla, Swerve, almond flour, and cheese.
3. Add blueberries and stir well.
4. Spray waffle maker with cooking spray.
5. Pour 1/4 batter in the hot waffle maker and cook for 8 minutes or until golden brown. Repeat with the remaining batter.
6. Serve and enjoy.

Nutrition:

Calories 96 Fat 6.1 carbohydrates 5.g Sugar 2.2 protein 6.1 cholesterol 86 mg

Super Easy Chocolate Chaffles

Preparation time: 10 minutes

Cooking Time: 5 minutes

Servings: 2

Ingredients:

- 1/4 cup unsweetened chocolate chips
- 1 egg
- 2 tbsps. almond flour
- 1/2 cup mozzarella cheese
- 1 tbsp. Greek yogurts
- 1/2 tsp. baking powder
- 1 tsp. stevia

Directions:

1. Switch on your square chaffle maker.
2. Spray the waffle maker with cooking spray.
3. Mix together all recipe ingredients in a mixing bowl.
4. Spoon batter in a greased waffle maker and make two chaffles.

5. Once chaffles are cooked, remove from the maker.
6. Serve with coconut cream, shredded chocolate, and nuts on top.
7. Enjoy!

Nutrition:

Protein: 35% 59 kcal Fat: 59% 99 kcal Carbohydrates: 6% 10 kcal

Cookies Chaffles

Preparation time: 6 minutes

Cooking Time: 5 minutes

Servings: 2

Ingredients:

- 1 egg
- 2 tbsps. almond flour
- 1 tbsp. peanut butter
- 1/2 tsp. baking powder
- 1 tsp. stevia
- 2 tbsps. cream cheese
- 2 tbsps. black cocoa powder
- 1 tbsp. mayonnaise
- 2 tbsps. chocolate chips

Directions:

1. In a small bowl, beat an egg with an electric beater.
2. Add the remaining ingredients and mix well until the batter is smooth and fluffy.

3. Divide the batter into portions.

4. Pour the batter in a minutes round greased waffle maker.

5. Cook Oreo chaffle cookies for about 2-3 minutes Utes until cooked.

6. Drizzle coconut flour on top.

7. Serve and enjoy!

Nutrition:

Protein: 22% 29 kcal Fat: 72% 96 kcal Carbohydrates: 7% 9 kcal

Yogurt Chaffle

Preparation time: 8 minutes

Cooking Time: 10 Minutes

Servings: 2

Ingredients:

- 1/2 cup mozzarella cheese, shredded
- 1/2 cup cheddar cheese, shredded
- 1 egg
- 2 tbsps. ground almonds
- 1 tsp. psyllium husk
- ¼ tsp. baking powder
- 1 tbsp. Greek yogurt

TOPPING

- 1 scoop heavy cream, frozen
- 1 scoop raspberry puree, frozen
- 2 raspberries

Directions:

1. Mix together all of the chaffle ingredients and heat up your Waffle Maker.
2. Let the batter stand for 5 minutes Utes.
3. Spray waffles maker with cooking spray.
4. Spread some cheese on chaffle maker and pour chaffle mixture in heart shape Belgian waffle maker.
5. Close the lid and cook for about 4-minutesutes.
6. For serving, scoop frozen cream and puree in the middle of chaffle.
7. Top with a raspberry.
8. Serve and enjoy!

Nutrition:

Protein: 31% 41 kcal Fat: 66% 88 kcal Carbohydrates: 3% 4 kcal

Brownie Chaffle

Preparation time: 5 minutes

Cooking Time:7–9 Minutes

Servings: 2

Ingredients:

Batter

- 4 eggs
- 4 ounces cottage cheese (½ cup)
- 1 teaspoon vanilla extract
- ¼ cup stevia
- ¼ cup melted butter
- ¼ cup almond flour
- 3 tablespoons cocoa powder
- ½ teaspoon baking powder

Other

- 2 tablespoons butter to brush the waffle maker
- 1 tablespoon cocoa powder for dusting
- ½ cup fresh raspberries for serving

Directions:

1. Preheat the waffle maker.
2. Add the eggs and cottage cheese to a bowl and stir in the vanilla extract, stevia, melted butter, almond flour, cocoa powder, and baking powder. Mix until just combined.
3. Brush the heated waffle maker with butter and add a few tablespoons of the batter.
4. Close the lid and cook for about 7–8 minutes depending on your waffle maker.
5. Serve with dusted cocoa powder and a few raspberries on top.

Nutrition:

Calories 281, fat 23.5 g, carbs 8.1 g, sugar 1.4 g, Protein 12.3 g, sodium 2 mg

Choco Waffle with Cream Cheese

Preparation time: 10 minutes

Cooking Time: 8 Minutes

Servings: 2

Ingredients:

Choco Chaffle

- 2 tablespoons cocoa powder
- 1 tablespoon almond flour
- ¼ teaspoon baking powder
- 2 tablespoons sweetener
- 1 egg, beaten
- ½ teaspoon vanilla extract
- 1 tablespoon heavy whipping cream

Frosting

- 2 tablespoons cream cheese
- 2 teaspoons confectioner's sugar (swerve)
- 1/8 teaspoon vanilla extract
- 1 teaspoon heavy cream

Directions:

1. Combine all the Choco chaffle ingredients in a large bowl, adding the wet ingredients last.
2. Mix well.
3. Plug in your waffle maker.
4. Pour half of the mixture into the device.
5. Close and cook for 4 minutes.
6. Cook the other waffle.
7. While waiting, make your frosting by adding cream cheese to a heat proof bowl.
8. Place in the microwave.
9. Microwave for 8 seconds.
10. Use a mixer to blend the cream cheese with the rest of the frosting ingredients.
11. Process until fluffy.
12. Spread the frosting on top of the chaffle.
13. Put another chaffle on top.
14. Pipe the rest of the frosting on top of the chaffle.
15. Slice and serve.

Nutrition: Calories 151 Total Fat 13 g Saturated Fat 6 g Cholesterol 111mg Sodium 83 mg Potassium 190 mg Total Carbohydrate 5 g Dietary Fiber 2 g Protein 6 g Total Sugars 1 g

Mini Keto Pizza

Preparation time: 10 minutes

Cooking Time: 15 Minutes

Servings: 2

Ingredients:

- 1 egg
- ½ cup mozzarella cheese, shredded
- ¼ teaspoon basil
- ¼ teaspoon garlic powder
- 1 tablespoon almond flour
- ½ teaspoon baking powder
- 2 tablespoons reduced-carb pasta sauce
- 2 tablespoons mozzarella cheese

Directions:

1. Preheat your waffle maker.
2. In a bowl, beat the egg.
3. Stir in the ½ cup mozzarella cheese, basil, garlic powder, almond flour and baking powder.

4. Add half of the mixture to your waffle maker.
5. Cook for 4 minutes.
6. Transfer to a baking sheet.
7. Cook the second mini pizza.
8. While both pizzas are on the baking sheet, spread the pasta sauce on top.
9. Sprinkle the cheese on top.
10. Bake in the oven until the cheese has melted.

Nutrition:

Calories 195 Total Fat 14 g Saturated Fat 6 g Cholesterol mg Sodium 301 mg Potassium 178 mg Total Carbohydrate 4 g Dietary Fiber 1 g Protein 13 g Total Sugars 1 g

Keto Chaffle With Almond Flour

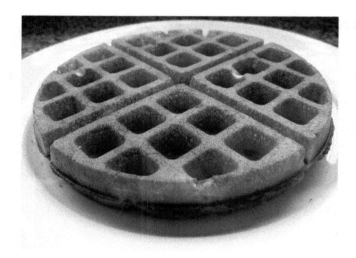

Preparation time: 10 minutes

Cooking Time: 8 Minutes

Servings: 2

Ingredients:

- 1 egg, beaten
- ½ cup cheddar cheese, shredded
- 1 tablespoon almond flour

Directions:

1. Turn on your waffle maker.
2. Mix all the ingredients in a bowl.
3. Pour half of the batter into the waffle maker.
4. Close the device and cook for minutes.
5. Remove from the waffle maker.
6. Let sit for 2 to 3 minutes.
7. Repeat the steps with the remaining batter.

Nutrition:

Calories 145 Total Fat 11 g Saturated Fat 7 g Cholesterol 112 mg Sodium 207 mg Potassium 15mg Total Carbohydrate 1 g Dietary Fiber 1 g Protein 10 g Total Sugars 1 g

Chaffles With Caramelized Apples and Yogurt

Preparation time: 10 minutes

Cooking Time: 10 Minutes

Servings: 2

Ingredients:

- 1 tablespoon unsalted butter
- 1 tablespoon golden brown sugar
- 1 Granny Smith apple, cored and thinly sliced
- 1 pinch salt
- 2 whole-grain frozen waffles, toasted
- 1/2 cup mozzarella cheese, shredded
- 1/4 cup Yoplait® Original French Vanilla yogurt Direction

Directions:

1. Melt the butter in a large skillet over medium-high heat until

2. starting to brown.

3. Add mozzarella cheese and stir well.

4. Add the sugar, apple slices and salt and cook, stirring frequently, until apples are softened and tender, about 6 to 9 minutes.

5. Put one warm waffle each on a plate, top each with yogurt and apples. Serve warm.

Nutrition:

Calories: 240 calories Total Fat: 10.4 g Cholesterol: 54 mg

Sodium: 226 mg Total Carbohydrate: 33.8 g Protein: 4.7 g

Peanut Butter Chaffle Cake

Preparation time: 10 minutes

Cooking Time: 10 Minutes

Servings: 2

Ingredients:

Chaffle

- 1 egg, beaten
- ¼ teaspoon baking powder
- 2 tablespoons peanut butter powder (sugar-free)
- ¼ teaspoon peanut butter extract
- 1 tablespoon heavy whipping cream
- 2 tablespoons sweetener

Frosting

- 2 tablespoons sweetener
- 1 tablespoon butter
- 1 tablespoon peanut butter (sugar-free)
- 2 tablespoons cream cheese
- ¼ teaspoon vanilla

Directions:

1. Preheat your waffle maker.
2. In a large bowl, combine all the ingredients for the chaffle.
3. Pour half of the mixture into the waffle maker.
4. Seal and cook for minutes.
5. Repeat steps to make the second chaffle.
6. While letting the chaffles cool, add the frosting ingredients in a bowl.
7. Use a mixer to turn mixture into fluffy frosting.
8. Spread the frosting on top of the chaffles and serve.

Nutrition:

Calories1 Total Fat 17 g Saturated Fat 8 g Cholesterol 97.1 mg Sodium 64.3 mg Potassium 342 mg Total Carbohydrate 3.6 g Dietary Fiber 0.6 g Protein 5.5 g Total Sugars 1.8 g

Keto Chaffle With Ice-cream

Preparation time: 10 minutes

Cooking Time: 5 Minutes

Servings: 2

Ingredients:

- 1 egg
- 1/2 cup cheddar cheese, shredded
- 1 tbsp. almond flour
- ½ tsp. baking powder.

FOR SERVING

- 1/2 cup heavy cream
- 1 tbsp. keto chocolate chips.
- 2 oz. raspberries
- 2 oz. blueberries

Directions:

1. Preheat your minutes waffle maker according to the manufacturer's instructions.
2. Mix together chaffle ingredients in a small bowl and make minutes chaffles.
3. For an ice-cream ball, mix cream and chocolate chips in a bowl and pour this mixture in 2 silicone molds.
4. Freeze the ice-cream balls in a freezer for about 2-hours.
5. For serving, set ice-cream ball on chaffle.
6. Top with berries and enjoy!

Nutrition:

Protein: 1 47 kcal Fat: 80% 219 kcal Carbohydrates: 3% 7 kcal

Chocolate Brownie Chaffles

Preparation time: 10 minutes

Cooking Time: 5 minutes

Servings: 2

Ingredients:

- 2 tbsp. cocoa powder
- 1 egg
- 1/4 tsp baking powder
- 1 tbsp. heavy whipping cream
- ½ cup mozzarella cheese

Directions:

1. Beat egg with a fork in a small mixing bowl.
2. Add the remaining ingredients in a beaten egg and beat well with a beater until the mixture is smooth and fluffy.
3. Pour batter in a greased preheated waffle maker.
4. Close the lid.
5. Cook chaffles for about 4 minutes Utes until they are thoroughly cooked.

6. Serve with berries and enjoy!

Nutrition:

Protein: 32% 51 kcal Fat: 62% 100 kcal Carbohydrates: 6% 10 kcal

Chaffle Tortilla

Preparation time: 10 minutes

Cooking Time: 8 Minutes

Servings: 2

Ingredients:

- 1 egg
- ½ cup cheddar cheese, shredded
- 1 teaspoon baking powder
- 4 tablespoons almond flour
- ¼ teaspoon garlic powder
- 1 tablespoon almond milk
- Homemade salsa
- Sour cream
- Jalapeno pepper, chopped

Directions:

1. Preheat your waffle maker.
2. Beat the egg in a bowl.

3. Stir in the cheese, baking powder, flour, garlic powder and almond milk.
4. Pour half of the batter into the waffle maker.
5. Cover and cook for 4 minutes.
6. Open and transfer to a plate. Let cool for 2 minutes.
7. Do the same for the remaining batter.
8. Top the waffle with salsa, sour cream and jalapeno pepper.
9. Roll the waffle.

Nutrition:

Calories 225 Total Fat 17.6g Saturated Fat 9.9g Cholesterol 117mg Sodium 367mg Potassium 366mg Total Carbohydrate 6g Dietary Fiber 0.8g Protein 11.3g Total Sugars 1.9g

Chicken Chaffle Sandwich

Preparation time: 10 minutes

Cooking Time: 15 Minutes

Servings: 2

Ingredients:

- 1 chicken breast fillet, sliced into strips
- Salt and pepper to taste
- 1 teaspoon dried rosemary
- 1 tablespoon olive oil
- 4 basic chaffles
- 2 tablespoons butter, melted
- 2 tablespoons Parmesan cheese, grated

Directions:

1. Season the chicken strips with salt, pepper and rosemary.
2. Add olive oil to a pan over medium low heat.
3. Cook the chicken until brown on both sides.
4. Spread butter on top of each chaffle.
5. Sprinkle cheese on top.

6. Place the chicken on top and top with another chaffle.

Nutrition:

Calories 262 Total Fat 20g Saturated Fat 9.2g Cholesterol mg Sodium 270mg Potassium 125mg Total Carbohydrate 1g Dietary Fiber 0.2g Protein 20.2g Total Sugars 0g

Chaffle With Cream Topping

Preparation time: 5 minutes

Cooking Time: 5minutes

Servings: 2

Ingredients:

- 1 cup egg whites
- ½ tsp. Vanilla
- 1 tsp. baking powder
- 1 cup mozzarella cheese, grated

TOPPING

- ½ cup frozen heavy cream
- Cherries

Directions:

1. Switch on your square waffle maker. Spray with non-stick spray.
2. Beat egg whites with beater, until fluffy and white.
3. Stir in the cheese, baking powder and vanilla.

4. Pour ½ of the batter in a waffle maker.

5. Close the maker and cook for about 3 minutes Utes.

6. Repeat with the remaining batter.

7. Remove chaffles from the maker.

8. Serve with heavy cream and cherries on top and enjoy!

Nutrition:

Protein: 38% 133 kcal Fat: 57% 201 kcal Carbohydrates: 5% 18 kcal

Chocolate Chip Chaffle

Preparation time: 10 minutes

Cooking Time: 8 Minutes

Servings: 2

Ingredients:

- 1 egg
- ½ teaspoon coconut flour
- ¼ teaspoon baking powder
- 1 teaspoon sweetener
- 1 tablespoon heavy whipping cream
- 1 tablespoon chocolate chips

Directions:

1. Preheat your waffle maker.
2. Beat the egg in a bowl.
3. Stir in the flour, baking powder, sweetener and cream.
4. Pour half of the mixture into the waffle maker.
5. Sprinkle the chocolate chips on top and close.
6. Cook for 4 minutes.

7. Remove the chaffle and put on a plate.
8. Do the same procedure with the remaining batter.

Nutrition:

Calories 146 Total Fat 10 g Saturated Fat 7 g Cholesterol 88 mg Sodium 140 mg Potassium 50 mg Total Carbohydrate 5 g Dietary Fiber 3 g Protein 6 g Total Sugars 1 g

Cheese Garlic Chaffle

Preparation time: 10 minutes

Cooking Time: 8 Minutes

Servings: 2

Ingredients:

Chaffle

- 1 egg
- 1 teaspoon cream cheese
- ½ cup mozzarella cheese, shredded
- ½ teaspoon garlic powder
- 1 teaspoon Italian seasoning

Topping

- 1 tablespoon butter
- ½ teaspoon garlic powder
- ½ teaspoon Italian seasoning
- 2 tablespoon mozzarella cheese, shredded

Directions:

1. Plug in your waffle maker to preheat.
2. Preheat your oven to 350 degrees F.
3. In a bowl, combine all the chaffle ingredients.
4. Cook in the waffle maker for minutes per chaffle.
5. Transfer to a baking pan.
6. Spread butter on top of each chaffle.
7. Sprinkle garlic powder and Italian seasoning on top.
8. Top with mozzarella cheese.
9. Bake until the cheese has melted.

Nutrition:

Calories141 Total Fat 13 g Saturated Fat 8 g Cholesterol 115.8 mg Sodium 255.8 mg Potassium 350 mg Total Carbohydrate 2.6g Dietary Fiber 0.7g

Cinnamon Cream Cheese Chaffle

Preparation time: 10 minutes

Cooking Time: 15 Minutes

Servings: 2

Ingredients:

- 2 eggs, lightly beaten
- 1 tsp collagen
- ¼ tsp baking powder, gluten-free
- 1 tsp monk fruit sweetener
- ½ tsp cinnamon
- ¼ cup cream cheese, softened
- Pinch of salt

Directions:

1. Preheat your waffle maker.
2. Add all ingredients into the bowl and beat using hand mixer until well combined.
3. Spray waffle maker with cooking spray.

4. Pour 1/2 batter in the hot waffle maker and cook for 3-minutes or until golden brown. Repeat with the remaining batter.
5. Serve and enjoy.

Nutrition:

Calories 179Fat 14.5 carbohydrates 1.9 sugar 0.4 protein 10.8 cholesterol 19mg

Lemon and Vanilla Chaffle

Preparation time: 5 minutes

Cooking Time:7–9 Minutes

Servings: 2

Ingredients:

Batter

- 4 eggs
- 4 ounces ricotta cheese
- 2 teaspoons vanilla extract
- 2 tablespoons fresh lemon juice
- Zest of ½ lemon
- 6 tablespoons stevia
- 5 tablespoons coconut flour
- ½ teaspoon baking powder

Other

- 2 tablespoons butter to brush the waffle maker

Directions:

1. Preheat the waffle maker.
2. Add the eggs and ricotta cheese to a bowl and stir with a wire whisk until just combined.
3. Add the vanilla extract, lemon juice, lemon zest, and stevia and mix until combined.
4. Stir in the coconut flour and baking powder until combined.
5. Brush the heated waffle maker with butter and add a few tablespoons of the batter.
6. Close the lid and cook for about 7–8 minutes depending on your waffle maker.
7. Serve and enjoy.

Nutrition:

Calories 200, fat 13.4 g, carbs 9 g, sugar 0.9 g, Protein 10.2 g, sodium 140 mg

Christmas Smoothie with Chaffles

Preparation time: 10 minutes

Cooking Time:0 Minutes

Servings: 2

Ingredients:

- 1 cup coconut milk
- 2 tbsps. almonds chopped
- ¼ cup cherries
- 1 pinch sea salt
- 1/4 cup ice cubes

FOR TOPPING

- 2 oz. keto chocolate chips
- 2 oz. cherries
- 2 minutes chaffles
- 2 scoop heavy cream, frozen

Directions:

1. Add almond milk, almonds, cherries, salt and ice in a blender, blend for 2 minutes Utes until smooth and fluffy.
2. Pour the smoothie into glasses.
3. Top with one scoop heavy cream, chocolate chips, cherries and chaffle in each glass.
4. Serve and enjoy!

Nutrition:

Protein: 4% 11 kcal Fat: 84% 24kcal Carbohydrates: 13% 37 kcal

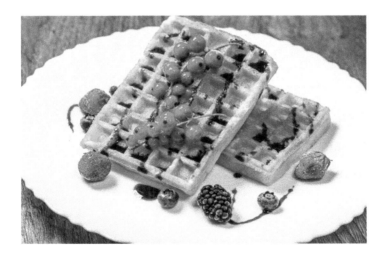

Raspberry and Chocolate Chaffle

Preparation time: 5 minutes

Cooking Time:7–9 Minutes

Servings: 2

Ingredients:

Batter

- 4 eggs
- 2 ounces cream cheese, softened
- 2 ounces sour cream
- 1 teaspoon vanilla extract
- 5 tablespoons almond flour
- ¼ cup cocoa powder
- 1½ teaspoons baking powder
- 2 ounces fresh or frozen raspberries

Other

- 2 tablespoons butter to brush the waffle maker
- Fresh sprigs of mint to garnish

Directions:

1. Preheat the waffle maker.
2. Add the eggs, cream cheese and sour cream to a bowl and stir with a wire whisk until just combined.
3. Add the vanilla extract and mix until combined.
4. Stir in the almond flour, cocoa powder, and baking powder and mix until combined.
5. Add the raspberries and stir until combined.
6. Brush the heated waffle maker with butter and add a few tablespoons of the batter.
7. Close the lid and cook for about 8 minutes depending on your waffle maker.
8. Serve with fresh sprigs of mint.

Nutrition:

Calories 270, fat 23 g, carbs 8.g, sugar 1.3 g, Protein 10.2 g,

sodium 158 mg

Keto Belgian Sugar Chaffles

Preparation time: 8 minutes

Cooking Time: 24 Minutes

Servings: 2

Ingredients:

- 1 egg, beaten
- 2 tbsp swerve brown sugar
- ½ tbsp butter, melted
- 1 tsp vanilla extract
- 1 cup finely grated Parmesan cheese

Directions:

1. Preheat the waffle iron.
2. Mix all the ingredients in a medium bowl.
3. Open the iron and pour in a quarter of the mixture. Close and cook until crispy, 6 minutes.
4. Remove the chaffle onto a plate and make 3 more with the remaining ingredients.

5. Cut each chaffle into wedges, plate, allow cooling and serve.

Nutrition:

Calories 13ats 9.45gCarbs 3.69gNet Carbs 3.69gProtein 8.5g

Pumpkin Chaffle With Maple Syrup

Preparation time: 10 minutes

Cooking Time: 16 Minutes

Servings: 2

Ingredients:

- 2 eggs, beaten
- ½ cup mozzarella cheese, shredded
- 1 teaspoon coconut flour
- ¾ teaspoon baking powder
- ¾ teaspoon pumpkin pie spice
- 2 teaspoons pureed pumpkin
- 4 teaspoons heavy whipping cream
- ½ teaspoon vanilla
- Pinch salt
- 2 teaspoons maple syrup (sugar-free)

Directions:

1. Turn your waffle maker on.
2. Mix all the ingredients except maple syrup in a large bowl.
3. Pour half of the batter into the waffle maker.
4. Close and cook for minutes.
5. Transfer to a plate to cool for 2 minutes.
6. Repeat the steps with the remaining mixture.
7. Drizzle the maple syrup on top of the chaffles before serving.

Nutrition:

Calories 201 Total Fat 15 g Saturated Fat g Cholesterol 200 mg Sodium 249 mg Potassium 271 mg Total Carbohydrate 4 g Dietary Fiber 1 g Protein 12 g Total Sugars 1 g

Maple Syrup & Vanilla Chaffle

Preparation time: 6 minutes

Cooking Time: 12 Minutes

Servings: 2

Ingredients:

- 1 egg, beaten
- ¼ cup mozzarella cheese, shredded
- 1 oz. cream cheese
- 1 teaspoon vanilla
- 1 tablespoon keto maple syrup
- 1 teaspoon sweetener
- 1 teaspoon baking powder
- 4 tablespoons almond flour

Directions:

1. Preheat your waffle maker.
2. Add all the ingredients to a bowl.
3. Mix well.
4. Pour some of the batter into the waffle maker.

5. Cover and cook for 4 minutes.

6. Transfer chaffle to a plate and let cool for 2 minutes.

7. Repeat the same process with the remaining mixture.

Nutrition:

Calories 146 Total Fat 9.5g Saturated Fat 4.3g Cholesterol 99mg Potassium 322mg Sodium 99mg Total Carbohydrate 10.6g Dietary Fiber 0.9g Protein 5.6g Total Sugars 6.4g

Sweet Vanilla Chocolate Chaffle

Preparation time: 10 minutes

Cooking Time: 10 Minutes

Servings: 2

Ingredients:

- 1 egg, lightly beaten
- 1/4 tsp cinnamon
- 1/2 tsp vanilla
- 1 tbsp Swerve
- 2 tsp unsweetened cocoa powder
- 1 tbsp coconut flour
- 2 oz cream cheese, softened

Directions:

1. Add all ingredients into the small bowl and mix until well combined.
2. Spray waffle maker with cooking spray.
3. Pour batter in the hot waffle maker and cook until golden brown.

4. Serve and enjoy.

Nutrition:

Calories 312 Fat 24 carbohydrates 11.5 sugar 0.8 protein 11.6 cholesterol 226 mg

Thanksgiving Keto Chaffles

Servings:5

Cooking Time:15minutes

Servings: 2

Ingredients:

- 4 oz. cheese, shredded
- 5 eggs
- 1 tsp. stevia
- 1 tsp baking powder
- 2 tsp vanilla extract
- 1/4 cup almond butter, melted
- 3 tbsps. almond milk
- 1 tsp avocado oil for greasing

Directions:

1. Crack eggs in a small mixing bowl; mix the eggs, almond flour, stevia, and baking powder.
2. Add the melted butter slowly to the flour mixture, mix well to ensure a smooth consistency.

3. Add the almond milk and vanilla to the flour and butter mixture, be sure to mix well.

4. Preheat waffles maker according to the manufacturer's instruction and grease it with avocado oil.

5. Pour the mixture into the waffle maker and cook until golden brown.

6. Dust coconut flour on chaffles and serve with coconut cream on the top.

Nutrition:

Protein: 3% 15 Kcal Fat: 94% 20Kcal Carbohydrates: 3% 15 Kcal

Garlic Cauliflower Chaffle

Preparation time: 10 minutes

Cooking Time: 8 Minutes

Servings: 2

Ingredients:

- 1 egg, beaten
- 1 cup cauliflower rice
- ½ cup cheddar cheese, shredded
- 1 teaspoon garlic powder

Directions:

1. Plug in your waffle maker.
2. Mix all the ingredients in a bowl.
3. Transfer half of the mixture to the waffle maker.
4. Close the device and cook for minutes.
5. Put the chaffle on a plate to cool for 2 minutes.
6. Repeat procedure to make the next chaffle.

Nutrition:

Calories 1 Total Fat 12.5g Saturated Fat 7g Cholesterol 112mg Sodium 267mg Total Carbohydrate 4.9g Dietary Fiber 0.1g Total Sugars 2.7g Protein 12g Potassium 73mg

Quick & Easy Blueberry Chaffle

Preparation time: 10 minutes

Cooking Time: 15 Minutes

Servings: 2

Ingredients:

- 1 egg, lightly beaten
- 1/4 cup blueberries
- 1/2 tsp vanilla
- 1 oz cream cheese
- 1/4 tsp baking powder, gluten-free
- 4 tsp Swerve
- 1 tbsp coconut flour

Directions:

1. Preheat your waffle maker.
2. In a small bowl, mix coconut flour, baking powder, and Swerve until well combined.
3. Add vanilla, cream cheese, egg, and vanilla and whisk until combined.

4. Spray waffle maker with cooking spray.
5. Pour half batter in the hot waffle maker and top with 4-blueberries and cook for 4-5 minutes until golden brown. Repeat with the remaining batter.
6. Serve and enjoy.

Nutrition:

Calories 135 Fat 8.2 carbohydrates 11 sugar 2.6 protein 5 cholesterol 9mg

Blueberry Chaffle

Preparation time: 10 minutes

Cooking Time: 8 Minutes

Servings: 2

Ingredients:

- 1 egg, beaten
- ½ cup mozzarella cheese, shredded
- 1 teaspoon baking powder
- 2 tablespoons almond flour
- 2 teaspoons sweetener
- ¼ cup blueberries, chopped

Directions:

1. Combine all the ingredients in a bowl. Mix well.
2. Turn on the waffle maker.
3. Pour half of the mixture into the cooking device.
4. Close it and cook for minutes.
5. Open the waffle maker and transfer to a plate.
6. Let cool for 2 minutes.

7. Add the remaining mixture to the waffle maker and repeat the steps.

Nutrition:

Calories 175 Total Fat 4.3g Saturated Fat 1.5g Cholesterol mg Sodium 76mg Potassium 296mg Total Carbohydrate 6.6g Dietary Fiber 1.7g Protein 5.3g Total Sugars 2g

Keto Smores Chaffle

Preparation Time: 5 minutes

Cooking Time: 10 minutes

Servings: 2

Ingredients:

- One large Egg
- ½ c. Mozzarella cheese shredded
- ½ tsp Vanilla extract
- Two tbs swerve brown
- ½ tbs Psyllium Husk Powder optional
- ¼ tsp Baking Powder
- Pinch of pink salt
- ¼ Lily's Original Dark Chocolate Bar
- Two tbs Keto Marshmallow Creme Fluff Recipe

Directions:

1. Make the batch of Keto Marshmallow Creme Fluff.
2. Whisk the egg until creamy.
3. Add vanilla and Swerve Brown, mix well.

4. Mix in the shredded cheese and blend.

5. Then add Psyllium Husk Powder, baking powder, and salt.

6. Mix until well incorporated, let the batter rest 3-4 minutes.

7. Prep/plug in your waffle maker to preheat.

8. Spread ½ batter on the waffle maker and cook 3-4 minutes.

9. Remove and set on a cooling rack.

10. Cook second half of batter same, then remove to cool.

11. Once cool, assemble the chaffless with the marshmallow fluff and chocolate: Using two tbs marshmallow and ¼ bar of Lily's Chocolate.

12. Eat as is, or toast for a melty and gooey Smore sandwich!

Nutrition: Calories: 0 Cal Total Fat: 8.1 g Saturated Fat: 0 g Cholesterol:111.2 mg Sodium: 1352.5 mg Total Carbs: 3.1 g Fiber: 0.2 g Sugar: 0.7g Protein: 8.3 g

Birthday Cake Chaffle

Preparation Time: 10 minutes

Cooking Time: 12 minutes

Servings: 2

Ingredients:

- 1 egg (beaten)
- 2 tbsp almond flour
- 1 tbsp swerve sweetener
- ½ tsp cake batter extract
- ¼ tsp baking powder
- 1 tbsp heavy whipping cream
- 2 tbsp cream cheese
- ½ tsp vanilla extract
- ½ tsp cinnamon

Frosting:

- 1 tbsp swerve
- ¼ cup heavy whipping cream
- ½ tsp vanilla extract

Directions:

1. Plug the waffle maker to preheat it and spray it with a non-stick spray.

2. In a mixing bowl, combine the cinnamon, almond flour, baking powder and swerve.

3. In another mixing bowl, whisk together the egg, vanilla, heavy cream, and cake batter extract.

4. Pour the flour mixture into the egg mixture and mix until the ingredients are well combined, and you have formed a smooth batter.

5. Pour an appropriate amount of the batter into the waffle maker and spread out the waffle maker to cover all the holes on the waffle maker.

6. Close the waffle maker and bake for about 3 minutes or according to your waffle maker's settings.

7. After the cooking cycle, use a silicone or plastic utensil to remove the chaffle from the waffle maker.

8. Repeat steps 5 to 7 until you have cooked all the batter into chaffless.

9. For the cream, whisk together the swerve, heavy cream and vanilla extract until smooth and fluffy.

10. To assemble the cake, place one chaffle on a flat surface and spread 1/3 of the cream over it. Layer another chaffle on the first one and spread 1/3 of the cream over it too.

11. Repeat this for the last chaffle and the remaining cream.

12. Cut cake and serve.

Nutrition:

Servings: 2 Amount per serving Calories 249 Daily Value Total Fat 23.1g 30% Saturated Fat 11.8g 59% Cholesterol 144mg 48% Sodium 75mg 3% Total Carbohydrate 6g 2% Dietary Fiber 1.1g 4% Total Sugars 0.8g Protein 5.8g Vitamin D 27mcg 136% Calcium 92mg 7% Iron 1mg 5% Potassium 139mg 3%

Strawberry Shortcake Chaffle

Preparation Time: 5 minutes

Cooking Time: 8 minutes

Servings: 2

Ingredients:

- ½ tsp cinnamon
- ½ cup shredded mozzarella cheese
- 1 tsp sugar free maple syrup
- 2 tsp granulated swerve
- 1 egg (beaten)
- 1 tbsp almond flour

Topping:

- 3 fresh strawberries (sliced)
- 2 tsp granulated swerve
- 1 tbsp heavy cream
- ¼ tsp vanilla extract
- 4 tbsp cream cheese (softened)

Directions:

1. Plug the waffle maker to preheat it and spray it with a non-stick cooking spray.
2. In a mixing bowl, combine the cinnamon, swerve, cheese and almond flour. Add the egg and maple syrup. Mix until the ingredients are well combined.
3. Close the waffle maker and cook for about 4 minutes or according to your waffle maker's settings4.   After the cooking cycle, remove the chaffle from the waffle maker with a plastic or silicone utensil.
4. Repeat steps 3 to 5 until you have cooked all the batter into chaffless.
5. For the topping, combine the cream cheese, swerve vanilla and heavy cream in a mixing bowl. Whisk until the mixture is smooth and fluffy.
6. Top the chaffless with the cream and sliced strawberries.
7. Serve and enjoy.

Nutrition:

Servings: 2 Amount per serving Calories 180% Daily Value Total Fat 15g 19% Saturated Fat 7.7g 38% Cholesterol 118mg 39% Sodium 137mg 6% Total Carbohydrate 5.2g 2%Dietary Fiber 1.1g 4% Total Sugars 1.3g Protein 7.3g Vitamin D 12mcg 58% Calcium 54mg 4% Iron 1mg 5% Potassium 90mg 2%

Carrot Cake Chaffle

Preparation Time: 10 minutes

Cooking Time: 18 minutes

Servings: 10 (6 mini chaffles)

Ingredients:

- 1 tbsp toasted pecans (chopped)
- 2 tbsp granulated swerve
- 1 tsp pumpkin spice
- 1 tsp baking powder
- ½ shredded carrots
- 2 tbsp butter (melted)
- 1 tsp cinnamon
- 1 tsp vanilla extract (optional)
- 2 tbsp heavy whipping cream
- ¾ cup almond flour
- 1 egg (beaten)

Butter cream cheese frosting:

- ½ cup cream cheese (softened)
- ¼ cup butter (softened)

- ½ tsp vanilla extract
- ¼ cup granulated swerve

Directions:

1. Plug the chaffle maker to preheat it and spray it with a non-stick cooking spray.
2. In a mixing bowl, combine the almond flour, cinnamon, carrot, pumpkin spice and swerve.
3. In another mixing bowl, whisk together the eggs, butter, heavy whipping cream, and vanilla extract.
4. Pour the flour mixture into the egg mixture and mix until you form a smooth batter.
5. Fold in the chopped pecans.
6. Close the waffle maker and cook for about 3 minutes or according to your waffle maker's settings.
7. After the cooking cycle, use a plastic or silicone utensil to remove the chaffle from the waffle maker.
8. Repeat steps 6 to 8 until you have cooked all the batter into chaffless.
9. For the frosting, combine the cream cheese and cutter int a mixer and mix until well combined.
10. Add the swerve and vanilla extract and slowly until the sweetener is well incorporated. Mix on high until the frosting is fluffy.

11. Place one chaffle on a flat surface and spread some cream frosting over it. Layer another chaffle over the first one a spread some cream over it too.

12. Repeat step 12 until you have assembled all the chaffless into a cake.

13. Cut and serve.

Nutrition:

Servings: 10 Amount per serving Calories 181 % Daily Value Total Fat 17.4g 22% Saturated Fat 8.1g 41% Cholesterol 52mg 17% Sodium 93mg 4% Total Carbohydrate 4.5g 2% Dietary Fiber 1.2g 4% Total Sugars0.6g Protein 3.5g Vitamin D 8mcg 39% Calcium 61mg 5% Iron 1mg4% Potassium 91mg 2%

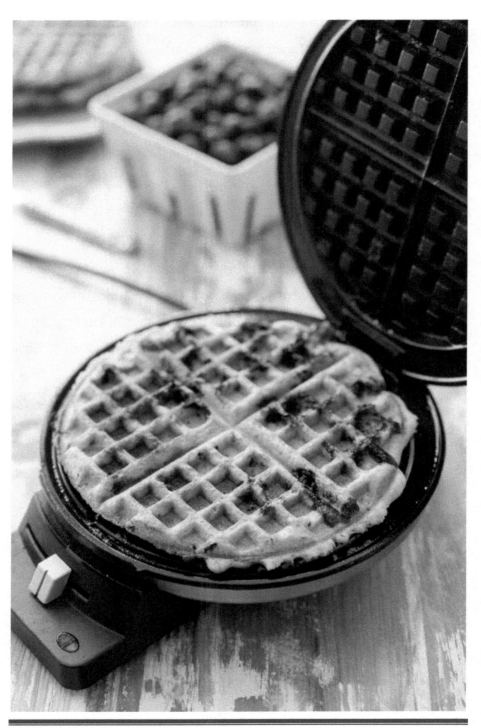

Lightning Source UK Ltd.
Milton Keynes UK
UKHW021306060521
383235UK00005B/94

9 781802 771619